YOUR KNOWLEDGE HAS VALUE

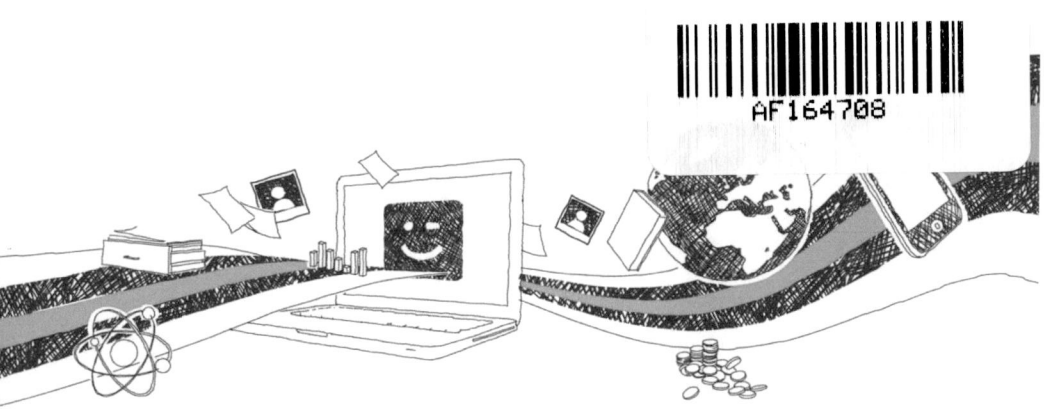

- We will publish your bachelor's and master's thesis, essays and papers

- Your own eBook and book - sold worldwide in all relevant shops

- Earn money with each sale

Upload your text at www.GRIN.com and publish for free

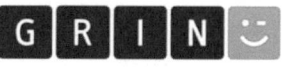

Bibliographic information published by the German National Library:

The German National Library lists this publication in the National Bibliography; detailed bibliographic data are available on the Internet at http://dnb.dnb.de .

This book is copyright material and must not be copied, reproduced, transferred, distributed, leased, licensed or publicly performed or used in any way except as specifically permitted in writing by the publishers, as allowed under the terms and conditions under which it was purchased or as strictly permitted by applicable copyright law. Any unauthorized distribution or use of this text may be a direct infringement of the author s and publisher s rights and those responsible may be liable in law accordingly.

Imprint:

Copyright © 2017 GRIN Verlag, Open Publishing GmbH
Print and binding: Books on Demand GmbH, Norderstedt Germany
ISBN: 9783668594210

This book at GRIN:

https://www.grin.com/document/384456

Patrick Kimuyu

Updates of the ACLS Guidelines 2015. A Historical Comparison

GRIN Publishing

GRIN - Your knowledge has value

Since its foundation in 1998, GRIN has specialized in publishing academic texts by students, college teachers and other academics as e-book and printed book. The website www.grin.com is an ideal platform for presenting term papers, final papers, scientific essays, dissertations and specialist books.

Visit us on the internet:

http://www.grin.com/

http://www.facebook.com/grincom

http://www.twitter.com/grin_com

Inhalt

Introduction 2
How the Phenomena Impacts Healthcare Delivery 2
How the Phenomena Impacts Nursing Care 3
Asystole and Pulseless Electrical Activity: Historical Context 4
Current Practice Guidelines for Asystole and Pulseless Electrical Activity 5
Ventricular Fibrillation and Pulseless Ventricular Tachycardia: Historical Context 6
Antiarrhythmics 7
2015 Guideline Updates 7
Amiodarone and Current ACLS Practice 8
Lidocaine 8
Implications of the Literature Review 9
Potential Research Questions 10
References 11

Introduction

Over the years, the American Heart Association has made outstanding contributions and numerous improvements to cardiopulmonary resuscitation and advanced cardiac life support guidelines. It is due to adequate use of resources and continuous research that millions of lives are saved in the United States. Such guidelines serve health care providers and other members of the healthcare team as a resource to ensure adequate and timely response to those individuals who experience cardiac or respiratory arrest. However, according to AHA statistics, "More than 326,000 people in the US suffer out-of-hospital cardiac arrests each year. Statistics prove that if more people knew CPR, more lives could be saved" (American Heart Association, 2016). In other words, dissemination of knowledge on the matter has direct outcomes on increasing survival rates. Therefore, the guidelines and the implementation methods are on continuous review based on new evidence. It is important to provide those who suffer cardiac or respiratory arrest with timely services because delays could end up affecting the outcome of those who experience reversible damage. Healthcare providers around the world have become informed on the benefits of updated competence and direct patient outcomes and quality of care. The American Heart Association has published the new 2015 cardiopulmonary resuscitation guidelines, where changes and updates are reflected in an effort to put the best available evidence in practice. The purpose of this review is to compare the 2015 AHA updates with historical evidence in an attempt to explicate the implications and limitations of pharmacology in advanced cardiac life support.

How the Phenomena Impacts Healthcare Delivery

Medical research and technology continue to open new doors for patients who are affected the most by clinical decision. In other words, knowledge about disease, medications, and interventions are no longer reserved for health professionals. Individuals can now seek to gain understanding through research. The Internet is one tool commonly used to help patients gain an understanding on his or her health condition and appropriate management. Therefore, each year there is more awareness on CPR and ACLS standards of practice for individuals and healthcare providers. The American Heart Association is a non-profit organization in the United States that uses research to reduce disability and deaths caused by cardiovascular disease and stroke.

The 2015 AHA guidelines on treating pulseless arrhythmia when promoting pressure support and return of spontaneous circulation pharmacologically have been reviewed and updated with the purpose of establishing one standard of care throughout the United States. The organization published updates on the recommended drugs to be used for asystole, pulseless electrical activity, ventricular fibrillation and pulseless ventricular tachycardia. The new changes will help promote effective treatment and return of spontaneous circulation. Therefore, it is essential for all members of the healthcare team to acquire the necessary skills, attitudes, communication, and appropiate resource utilization to help obtain positive patient experience and outcomes.

How the Phenomena Impacts Nursing Care

Over the years, The American Heart Association has taken part in the development of measures to help ensure timely and accurate treatment and interventions for those who experience cardiac or respiratory arrest. By having a clear understanding of the guidelines on basic life support and advanced cardiac life support the nurse can build a strong foundation on tested evidence. Leading to improved patient outcomes in acute and non-acute care settings. Nursing is not a profession that can be defined easily because it is variable in nature. A nurse is the person most involved in the care of those experiencing a difficult time in their health. Nursing is also a profession that focuses on the care of all individuals within the community. However, in order to maintain professionalism in patient care it is essential to follow the code of ethics. As demonstrated in the A.H.A 2015 updates, ethics is greatly emphasized during critical decision periods.

By following the code of ethics and principles highlighted in the AHA updates, health care providers can make educated decisions with a foundation in positive patient outcomes. One of the most important rules that guide the nurse's professional practice is the "Do no harm" principle. This principle serves physicians and nurses as a guide to primarily consider the patient's well being above all. As stated by the American Nurses Association, "Clear, accurate, and accessible information is an essential element of safe, quality, evidence-based nursing practice" (2014, para 2). In an attempt to maintain clarity, the AHA created algorhythms to help increase patient safety, promote better inter-professional communication and prevent delay of care in the general population and acute care settings.

Today, being able to refer to A.H.A guidelines is a tremendous advantage that many countries around the world lack. The guide is detailed and specifically tailored to the incidences of cardiac arrests in the United States and at the same time is setting driven. As stated in the update, there are now two separate algorithms for cardiac quality cardiopulmonary resuscitation. The algorithm for non-healthcare personnel is a basic approach to cardiopulmonary resuscitation and life support. All individuals are encouraged to become familiar with the basic course of action that a non-HCP personnel rescuer should perform for life support.

Asystole and Pulseless Electrical Activity: Historical Context

Asystole and Pulseless Electrical Activity (PEA) are the two non-shockable rhythms. Therefore, ACLS providers focus more on identifying primary cause, performing CPR, and administering epinephrine. However, over the years the American heart Association has contributed with specific guidelines that are based on research. Such guidelines have been updated twice in the past six years, 2010 and 2015. In the A.H.A 2010 guidelines, the use of Epinephrine and Vasopressin is recommended along with other medications aiming to treat the specific cause of the PEA. As highlighted in the 2010 book guidelines, epinephrine 1 mg IV/IO is administered every 3-5 minutes with an option to change the first or second dose of epinephrine for Vasopressin 40 mg IV/IO (American Heart Association, 2011). The 2010 CPR and ACLS manual also states that asystole often represents an agonal rhythm confirming death, rather than a rhythm to be treated. It is for the same reason that cardiac defibrillation is not recommended.

An article written by Todd A. Miano, Pharm.D and Michael A. Crouch, Pharm. D on the role of Vasopressin in the treatment of cardiac arrest was reviewed. It states that vasopressin like Epinephrine is effective promoting peripheral vasoconstriction, an essential goal when treating cardiac arrest patients. However, Vasopressin dilates cerebral blood vessels, improving cerebral perfusion during cardiac arrest (Miano & Crouch, 2006). By doing so patients can experience less neurologic deficits upon return of spontaneous circulation. The research also highlights that Vasopressin can be effective in treating hypoxia and metabolic acidosis for patients with prolonged cardiac arrests. Another point mentioned in the article is that when compared to Epinephrine, Vasopressin has a longer half-life of 10 to 20 minutes (Miano & Crouch, 2006). The article notes that Vasopressin is studied in animal models in contrast to Epinephrine in animal and in vitro studies. According to Miano and Crouch, for the first time the updated 2005 AHA guidelines suggested one dose of vasopressin 40 units may be given intravenously or intraosseous to replace the first or second dose of epinephrine in all pulseless cardiac arrests (Miano & Crouch, 2006). An identified cofounding variable in the article was that patients studied had received both epinephrine and Vasopressin. Therefore, there was no isolated study for Vasopressin.

Current Practice Guidelines for Asystole and Pulseless Electrical Activity

According to the official website for the 2015 American Heart Association recommendations and updates for cardiopulmonary resuscitation measures are based on an "[e]xtensive evidence review process that was begun by the International Liaison Committee on Resuscitation after the publication of the International Liaison Committee on Resuscitation (ILCOR) 2010 completed in February 2015" (2016, para 3). The 2015 recommendations for asystole and pulseless electrical activity when the rhythm check reveals a non-shockable rhythm, is to begin chest compressions, and continue CPR for two minutes before the rhythm check is repeated.

Administration of Epinephrine as soon as possible after the onset of cardiac arrest continues to be the initial treatment for a non-shockable rhythm. It is because a large observational study compared Epinephrine given at one to three minutes with Epinephrine given at three later time intervals (American Heart Association, 2016). The study was able to conclude that a positive relationship existed between early administration of Epinephrine and increased return of spontaneous circulation, with increased percentages of survival to hospital discharge, and neurologically intact survival. In contrast, according to a systematic review and meta-analysis created by Koko Ang, MD, MPH; and Thwe Htay, MD regarding the use of vasopressin for cardiac arrest concluded that, "[t]here is no clear advantage of vasopressin over epinephrine in the treatment of cardiac arrest. Guidelines for Advanced Cardiac Life Support should not recommend vasopressin in resuscitation protocols until more solid human data on its superiority are available" (Koko Aung & Thwe Htay, 2005). The AHA has also concluded that when Vasopressin is administered as a substitute for the first or second dose of epinephrine no advantages were discovered. Therefore, Vasopressin has been removed from the algorithm in an attempt to keep simplicity and clarity.

A literature review with the goal of identifying the standard of practice for treating asystole and or pulseless electrical activity pulseless arrhythmias when promoting pressure support and return of spontaneous circulation pharmacologically, has been conducted. A non-randomized study was found in reference to the use of Epinephrine as the first line of treatment for asystole and or pulseless electrical activity. An article published by Clifton W. Callaway, MD, PhD for the University of Pittsburgh, focused on the implications of epinephrine as the primary drug administered to reverse cardiac arrest. Callaway (2013) states that dose, timing, and indications for epinephrine use are based on limited animal data and recent studies question whether Epinephrine provides any overall benefit for patients. The available clinical data suggested that epinephrine administered during CPR could increase short-term survival, but would not benefit or harm patients in the long-term or affect functional recovery (Clifton W. Callaway, 2013). In other words, the author implies that the longer the patient remains in asystole the higher the dose of total Epinephrine. The results of the studies correlate increased Epinephrine dosages with negative neurological outcome upon return of circulation and reductions of microvascular blood flow despite macroscopic increases in perfusion pressures (Clifton W. Callaway, 2013). The implications for patients can be more harming than beneficial for long-term quality of life, creating and ethical dilemma. In addition, the total dose of Epinephrine administered is proportional to how long a patient remains in cardiac arrest, resulting in higher doses for patients who fail to respond to initial treatment. Therefore, adverse relationship between Epinephrine dose and outcome is largely attributed to systematic bias in study design (Clifton W. Callaway, 2013). The conclusion states that more trials are needed. In addition, according to a systematic review and meta-analysis done by Ignacio Morales, MD; Maria Del Rocio Valverde-Leon, MD; and Maria Aurora Rodriguez-Borrego, MD; regarding the use of epinephrine in cardiac arrest concluded that "administration of epinephrine appears to increase the rate of ROSC, but when compared with other therapies, no positive effect was found on survival rates of patients with favorable neurological status" (Ignacio Morales, Maria Del Rocio Valverde-Leon, & and Maria Aurora Rodriguez-Borrego, 2016).

Ventricular Fibrillation and Pulseless Ventricular Tachycardia: Historical Context

Pulseless ventricular fibrillation is a shockable rhythm caused an abnormality in the electrical conduction system of the heart. According to the American Heart Association 2010 guidelines, electrical defibrillation is the most effective way to treat ventricular fibrillation. It is also the priority in promoting survival after cardiac arrest, since v-fib turns to asystole if not treated rapidly. The 2010 guidelines highlight that the initial action with ventricular fibrillation and ventricular tachycardia is to deliver shock, resume chest compressions, and go about two cycles of CPR (American Heart Association, 2011). The AHA 2010 guide also includes important drugs utilized to reverse ventricular fibrillation and ventricular tachycardia known as antiarrhyhtmics. The guide recommends to administer amiodarone or lidocaine before or after delivering the shock.

Antiarrhythmics

The 2010 ACLS guide promotes the use of Amiodarone as the first line antiarrhythmic. The guide states that it has been clinically demonstrated that Amiodarone improves the rate of return of spontaneous circulation in adults with refractory VF/ pulseless VT. They recommend amiodarone 300 mg IV/IO bolus, then a second additional dose of 150 mg IV/IO once. If Amiodarone is not available, Lidocaine may be administered at 1-1.5 mg/kg IV/IO first dose then 0.5-0.75 mg/kg IV/IO at 5-10 minutes intervals, to a max dose of 3mg/kg. According to the AHA Lidocaine has no proven short-term or long-term favorable outcome. Even if lidocaine lacks proven results, it is considered an alternative antiarrhythmic in an attempt to save a life (American Heart Association, 2011).

2015 Guideline Updates

The official 2010 American Heart Association guidelines for ACLS have been updated in 2015. The new protocol has discontinued vasopressin as the alternative to the first or second dose to Epinephrine in the algorithm. The guidelines also highlight that CPR should be resumed immediately after shock delivery without a rhythm or pulse check, and continue with chest compressions for two minutes before the next rhythm check. In addition, Amiodarone remains the antiarrhythmic of choice for VF/pVT unresponsive to CPR, defibrillation, and Epinephrine. While Lidocaine is still considered as an alternative to amiodarone there is ongoing research on survival and neurologic outcomes (American Heart Association, 2016).

Amiodarone and Current ACLS Practice

An experimental swine model study was conducted in 2014 by the Department of Internal Medicine in a hospital in Athens, Greece. The study aimed to compare hemodynamic effects and outcomes with early administration of amiodarone and epinephrine versus epinephrine alone in pigs with prolonged ventricular fibrillation (VF) (Karlis, 2014). They randomly administered bolus doses of epinephrine 0.02 mg/kg and either amiodarone (5mg/kg) or saline after 8 minutes of untreated VF arrest. Cardiopulmonary resuscitation CPR was inititated immediately after drug administration and defibrillation was attempted 2 minutes later. CPR was resumed for another 2 minutes after each defibrillation attempt, and the same dose of epinephrine was given every 4th minute during CPR. Haemodynamic monitoring continued for 6 hours after return of spontaneous circulation (ROSC). The results of the study showed no difference in rates of ROSC and 48 hour survival with amiodarone vs saline. The study concluded that early administration of amiodarone did not imrpove ROSC or 48 hr survival rate, and was associated with worse haemodynamics in this swine model of cardiac arrest (Karlis, 2014).

Lidocaine

The American Heart Association 2015 Advanced Cardiac Life Support Guidelines still consider lidocaine as an alternative to amiodarone when treating ventricular fibrillation and or pulseless ventricular tachycardia. A randomized double blinded control trial study conducted in the University of Medical Sciences in Tehran, Iran was reviewed. The study aimed to evaluate the effectiveness of single dose of amiodarone or lidocaine by the way of pump circuit 3 minutes before aortic cross clamp release and compare the results with normal saline as placebo.. The methodology used in the study involved 150 patients scheduled for first time elective coronary artery bypass graft surgery were randomly assigned to receive either single dose of amiodarone (150 mg), lidocaine (100 mg), or normal saline (5 ml) 3 minutes before aortic cross clamp release The incidence of ventricular fibrillation was higher in the placebo group (15.9%) when compared to Lidocaine (11.8%) and Amiodarone (8.9%).No statistical difference among the three groups was found. However the reuse of Amiodarone was statistically greater than Lidocaine (Alireza Alizadeh-Ghavidel, 2013). The implication for practice of Lidocaine is important for current AHA guidelines in terms of implementing Amiodarone before Lidocaine. The AHA continues to further research the use of Lidocaine as the first line antiarrhythmic. Currently, the AHA recommends hospital and acute care settings to implement the 2015 guidelines as soon as possible (American Heart Association, 2016).

Implications of the Literature Review

When concluding the information gathered the researcher can appreciate how the American Heart Association and other important health care identities implement extensive research in the interest of wellness. Moreover, in order to help disseminate the best evidence available on cardiopulmonary resuscitation a variety of resources are available at no cost. The AHA promotes awareness not only for healthcare providers but for those individuals with limited knowledge on CPR. The AHA creates visual aids, videos, and algorithms to help remember important steps of the chain of survival. The resources reviewed highlight the latest evidence available with regards to standards of practice for treating asystole and or pulseless electrical activity pulseless arrhythmias when promoting pressure support and return of spontaneous circulation pharmacologically. Being competent on the updates assures that health care providers who practice in acute care settings primarily, provide one single standard of care. Pharmacology plays an important role in increasing the incidence of survival and return of spontaneous circulation and preventing death. Therefore, reviewing the importance and benefits of each drug class will help the provider make wise decisions on treatment for the specific case.

Moving forward with the information gathered health care providers could contribute to better patient outcomes by implementing patient specific treatment and conscientious use of the guidelines. An essential part of moving forward with the current evidence is creating studies in hospitals and evaluating outcomes in units such as acute coronary care and stroke units. Promoting further education of health providers would ensure best practice, for instance by utilizing simulation of scenarios. Moreover, further research needs to be conducted in health care settings with high rates of cardiac arrest as well as low survival upon hospital discharge statistics. Being able to identify the places that are providing poor interventions can serve as a resource for improvement.

Potential Research Questions

The purpose of the literature review is to compare and contrast the 2015 AHA updates with historical evidence in an attempt to explicate the implications and limitations of pharmacology in advanced cardiac life support. The evidence reviewed indicates that future research needs to concentrate on setting specific issues related to the treatment of cardiac arrests. The 2015 American Heart Association guidelines have concentrated on simplicity with the purpose of emphasizing the importance of compressions and early implementation of algorithms, defibrillation and medication administration. However, more emphasis is needed in the area of long term outcomes and use of the emergency medications. Most of the sources reviewed attempt to prove how vasopressors and antiarrhythmic fail to provide long term outcomes after administration. Moreover, the resources reviewed are often used by health care providers but fail to translate the audience the relevance and implications of utilizing the results in patient care. Some questions the nurse researcher developed after connecting the current evidence are:

What are long term effects of Epinephrine, Amiodarone, and Lidocaine administration?

Dose safety and bioaccumulation leading to organ failure within the first 48 hours period post return of spontaneous circulation?

Effects of Epinephrine, Amiodarone , and Lidocaine on neurologic functions after hospital discharge?

Preventing cardiac arrest in patients at high risks with chronic diseases such as heart failure, diabetes, and kidney disease? Early recognition of signs and symptoms that put patients at risk for cardiac arrest.

References

Alireza Alizadeh-Ghavidel, S. N. (2013). Amiodarone versus lidocaine for the prevention of reperfusion ventricular fibrillation: A randomized clinical trial. *Arya Atherosclerosis*, 343–349.

American Heart Association. (2011). *Advanced Cardiovascular Life Support.* Dallas: American Heart Association.

American Heart Association. (2016). *American Heart Association.* Retrieved from American Heart Association: http://www.heart.org/HEARTORG/CPRAndECC/CPR_UCM_001118_SubHomePage.js

American Nurses Association. (2014, (n.d.) (n.d.)). *What is Nursing?* Retrieved from American Nurses Association: http://www.nursingworld.org/especiallyforyou/what-is-nursing

Clifton W. Callaway, M. P. (2013). Epinephrine forCardiac Arrest. *Current Opinion in Cardiology*, 36–42.

G. Karlis, N. I. (2014). Effects of early amiodarone administration during and immediately aftercardiopulmonary resuscitation in swine model. *Acta Anaesthesiologica*

Ignacio Morales, M., Maria Del Rocio Valverde-Leon, M., & Maria Aurora Rodriguez-Borrego, M. (2016). Epinephrine in Cardiac Arrest: Systematic Review and Meta-Analysis. *Revista Latino-Americana de Enfermagem*, 24.

Scandinavica, 114–122.

Koko Aung, M., & Thwe Htay, M. (2005, January 10). Vasopressin for Cardiac Arrest a Systematic Review and Meta Analysis. *Arch Intern Med*, 165:17-24.

Miano, T. A., & Crouch, M. A. (2006). Evolving Role of Vasopressin in the Treatment of Cardiac Arrest. *Pharmacotherapy: The Journal of Human Pharmacology and Drug Therapy*, 838-839.

XIAO-LI, J., DONG-PING, W., XIN, L., HUI, L., XIAO-XING, L., YAN, X., & XI-FU, W. (2010). Vasopressin and epinephrine versus epinephrine in management of patients with cardiac arrest: a meta-analysis. *Signa Vitae*, 5(1), 20-26.

YOUR KNOWLEDGE HAS VALUE

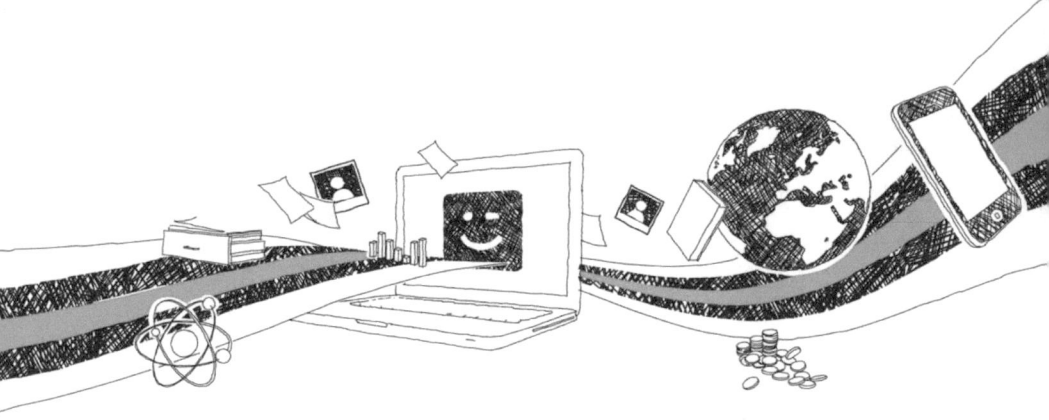

- We will publish your bachelor's and master's thesis, essays and papers

- Your own eBook and book - sold worldwide in all relevant shops

- Earn money with each sale

Upload your text at www.GRIN.com and publish for free

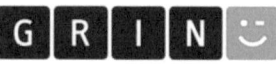